TARA JAMES

Fashion Therapy: A Guide to Finding Your Personal Style

First edition

This book was professionally typeset on Reedsy.
Find out more at reedsy.com

Contents

1

Introduction

First things first, this book isn't about retail therapy. This book will not be encouraging you to shop till you drop, but it will help you to build a wardrobe that will make you feel like the best version of your best self.

Before you start this book you need the following:

- A wardrobe that needs refining.
- A body to dress.
- A notebook and pen to take notes and complete the tasks given throughout the book to help you identify your personal style.

By the time you finish this book, you will be best friends with your personal style and your wardrobe will feel like a healthier space.

2

Establishing Your Personal Style

Fashion holds significant importance in society for various reasons. One of the most prominent aspects of fashion is its role in self-expression. The way individuals dress and present themselves can serve as a powerful means of conveying their unique identities, personalities, and values. From choosing certain colours and patterns to accessorising, fashion enables people to communicate aspects of their inner selves without saying a word. Throwback to when you were little and would dress up your dolls for fun, but now you can do this with yourself and your life-size wardrobe.

Fashion's influence extends beyond the material realm, impacting individuals psychologically. Studies have shown that what we wear can affect our mood and behaviour; this is an amazing concept called "enclothed cognition." The clothes we choose can shape our cognitive processes, influencing our thoughts and the way we act and even affecting our confidence and self-esteem. When we put on specific types of clothing, we tend to adopt the associated psychological traits and characteristics linked to those garments. For example, wearing a professional suit might make us feel more confident, competent, and authoritative, leading us to perform better on work-related tasks. On the other hand, donning casual and comfortable clothing might promote a relaxed and approachable demeanour, making social interactions more enjoyable. We have all heard the saying 'dress to impress', we should implement this into our real lives, but only to impress ourselves in order to feel fashionably fabulous. You have the ability to curate the perfect wardrobe that makes you feel how you want to feel every time you get dressed. Knowing this in itself can be very therapeutic in the sense that you can essentially be anyone you want to be if you simply dress the part.

Enclothed cognition can influence our mood and emotional state. Wearing clothes that we perceive as aesthetically pleasing or that hold positive memories can uplift our spirits and create a sense of well-being within. Conversely, wearing uncomfortable or ill-fitting clothes might lead to feelings of distress and discomfort, negatively affecting our overall emotional experience.

This phenomenon also extends to the concept of "dressing for success." The idea is that by dressing in a manner associated with success and achievement, individuals can enhance their motivation and performance in various tasks. For example, if you wear a suit for a job interview or a nice dress on a date, you feel like you are more likely to win the job, or the man. The confidence and self-assuredness that come with wearing appropriate and empowering clothing can lead to improved focus and even better productivity.

Fashion serves as a form of self-expression and creativity, a reflection of culture as well as history, and a means of influencing social and professional impressions, even if we aren't totally aware of this when we get dressed. By embracing fashion and style, individuals can find empowerment, connect with their cultural roots, and engage in an ever-evolving art form that shapes our society and individual identities.

Personal style and enclothed cognition are closely connected concepts that demonstrate how our clothing choices not only reflect our identity but also influence our thoughts, emotions, and behaviour. Personal style refers to the unique way individuals choose to express themselves through clothing, reflecting their preferences, values, and personality traits. Enclothed cognition, as discussed earlier, is a psychological phenomenon where the clothes we wear impact our cognitive processes and emotional experiences. This is why it is so important to ensure we dress for ourselves and have a wardrobe that reflects our personal style.

Personal style is an essential aspect of how anyone chooses to present themselves to the world. It goes beyond merely following fashion trends that we all see in magazines and on our social media feeds and delves into the realm of self-expression, identity, and creativity (it is not as scary as it sounds).

At its core, personal style is about authenticity and individuality. It allows us to showcase our true selves and embrace what makes us unique. Each person's personal style is a reflection of themselves, making it a powerful tool for self-discovery and self-awareness.

For some, personal style is a canvas for artistic expression. They use clothing as a means to create wearable art, experimenting with colours, patterns, and silhouettes to make a bold statement about who they are and what they stand for. Others will use a minimalistic and timeless approach, choosing classic and understated pieces. This book will not force you to opt for either; you just need to ensure you are being true to yourself and honest with what you like. It doesn't matter what you have seen everyone else wearing on social media or what is 'trendy' right now; it matters that you feel your best self in the clothes that you are wearing.

An important rule to remember is that personal style is not stagnant; like anything in life, personal style evolves and adapts with us as we grow and change. As we go through various stages of life, our style may transform to reflect our shifting priorities and aspirations. Most of us have been through a boho or grungy phase. This may be embarrassing to look back on now, but that fashion phase has allowed you to develop an understanding of what you do and don't feel comfortable wearing.

Emotional significance plays a significant role in personal style; hence, it can link to your overall well-being. Certain clothes may hold sentimental value, reminding us of important events, loved ones, or cherished memories. Wearing these pieces can evoke feelings of nostalgia and comfort, providing a sense of connection to the past and a source of emotional support. This is often overlooked in today's world of fast fashion (which we will discuss later on). Some of the hero items in your wardrobe could be passed down as heirlooms from family members. For example, a grandmother's engagement ring could hold significant emotional value for the individual who owns it.

Moreover, personal style is intrinsically tied to confidence and self-esteem. When we dress in a way that aligns with our self-perception and makes us feel good about ourselves, our confidence soars. What more could you want? The right outfit can boost our mood, elevate our posture, and even enhance our performance in various areas of life. This is how magical the power of dressing can be! We should all keep this in mind when we are curating our wardrobes and getting dressed every morning.

While personal style is deeply individual, it can also serve as a form of social communication. Clothing choices convey messages and signals about our values, interests, and social affiliations. Your look could create an initial impression on others, influencing how you are perceived and treated. For example, wearing a flowing light pink dress could create a particular impression that is often associated with femininity, grace, and a relaxed, carefree attitude. Let's be honest; we have all made assumptions about people based on their outfits.

One of the most significant aspects of personal style is that it is a conscious choice. We have the freedom to curate our wardrobes and experiment with different looks until we find the ones that resonate most with our inner selves. Later in this book, you will be given activities to allow yourself to become more conscious of what your personal style actually is and to make conscious choices when it comes to your wardrobe.

Personal style is not about conforming to external standards or seeking validation from others; it is about cultivating a deep sense of self-acceptance and self-love. When we dress in a way that feels authentic and aligned with our true selves, we radiate a magnetic energy that draws people towards us.

In summary, personal style is a powerful means of self-expression, creativity, and empowerment. It is an ever-evolving journey of self-discovery, allowing us to communicate who we are without uttering a word. By embracing our personal style, we honour our individuality, celebrate our uniqueness, and harness the transformative power of clothing to uplift ourselves and inspire those around us.

Finding your personal style is an exciting journey of self-discovery and self-expression. Creating the perfect wardrobe for yourself involves a combination of self-awareness, exploration, and a selective approach to curating your clothing collection. So what are we waiting for? Let's get to the fun part and start exploring your personal style.

Activity 1

With the following 5 categories, create a list of things that instantly come to mind. Do this brainstorming activity without overthinking each category to get a raw view of what your personal style is really craving.

*1. **Silhouettes:** What are your favourite types of wardrobe silhouettes? Understanding different silhouettes can help you choose clothing that complements your body shape and expresses your personal style. Write down which ones you like and dislike. If you are not sure what silhouettes suit you, take yourself to the mall and* *experiment in the changing room. Consider the following shapes:*

Maxi: The maxi silhouette involves long, flowing garments that reach down to the ankles or floor, creating an elongated and elegant look.

Crop: A crop silhouette features shorter tops, jackets, or pants, exposing a portion of the midriff or ankles.

Oversized: The oversized silhouette involves loose and baggy clothing, providing a comfortable and relaxed style.

Boxy: This silhouette has a more structured, square shape, often seen in boxy tops or jackets.

A-line: This silhouette is characterised by a fitted bodice that gradually flares out from the waist down in the shape of the letter "A." A-line dresses and skirts are versatile and flattering on many body types.

Fit-and-Flare: Similar to the A-line, this silhouette has a fitted bodice but flares out dramatically from the waist, creating a more pronounced "flared" effect.

Hourglass: This silhouette emphasises the natural curves of the body, with a well-defined waist and balanced proportions between the bust and hips.

Empire: The empire silhouette features a high waistline just below the bust, with a loose and flowing skirt that falls gracefully over the hips and waist.

Peplum: This silhouette incorporates a short overskirt or ruffles that flares out from the waist, often adding volume and visual interest to dresses, tops, or jackets.

Bell-shaped: A bell-shaped silhouette is characterised by a fitted bodice and a skirt that gradually flares out, resembling the shape of a bell.

Balloon: This silhouette involves voluminous fabric gathered at the waist or hip and then tapering down to create a "balloon" effect.

Trapeze: A trapeze silhouette features a flared and swingy shape, usually beginning with a fitted neckline and gradually widening towards the hem.

Flapper: This is a popular 1920s silhouette that is characterised by its straight and loose shape, often accompanied by dropped waistlines and fringed details.

Pencil: A pencil silhouette is narrow and form-fitting, typically seen in skirts or dresses that follow the contours of the body.

2. Statement pieces *- Do you currently have any favourite statement pieces? Or have you seen any celebrities rocking cool pieces that you have loved? Wardrobe statement pieces are standout items that add a unique and eye-catching element to your looks. These key pieces often reflect your personal style and can elevate an entire look. Here are just some different types of wardrobe statement pieces you can consider:*

Statement Earrings: Oversized or intricate statement earrings draw attention to your face and can be the focal point of your outfit. You could consider metals, pearls, or sparkles.

Unique Sunglasses: A pair of trendy or quirky sunglasses can add a playful and fashionable touch to your overall look. From cat eyes, to aviators, there is so much choice.

A fun Jacket: From a classic leather jacket that instantly adds edge to an oversized bomber, or a fun jacket can dress up (or down) a simple look like jeans and a white top.

Statement Handbag: An eye-catching handbag in a unique shape, cool colour, or crazy pattern can instantly elevate your ensemble and show off your fashion sense.

Colourful Coat: A brightly coloured or patterned coat can make a bold statement during the colder months. A coat is often the most seen piece of clothing during the winter, so it is worth investing in.

Chunky Statement Necklace: A chunky, attention-grabbing necklace can instantly transform a basic outfit into a stylish and polished ensemble. This could be a chunky chain or a pretty pendant.

Patterned Scarf: A colourful or intricately patterned scarf can be a versatile accessory to tie together an outfit and add visual interest. A silk scarf can add some class to a summer wardrobe, and a thick knitted scarf can add a warm, cosy feel to a winter outfit.

*3. **Dislikes** - What pieces in your wardrobe do you not like? Fashion dislikes can be highly subjective and vary from person to person. What one individual dislikes, another might love, so this brainstorm may be slightly harder. You may love a certain look or piece on someone else, but not feel comfortable in that particular style yourself. Jot all of these things down. Ultimately, it's essential to wear clothing that makes you feel comfortable and confident, regardless of prevailing trends or popular opinions.*

*4. **Colours**- What colours make you feel amazing when you are wearing them? Fashion colours can change with each season and evolving trends. However, some favourites will stand the test of time and continue to be popular in your wardrobe. Which of the following colours do you love? Think of the connotations of each of the colours and what vibe you want to give off.*

Black: Classic and versatile, black is a staple in many wardrobes (but don't feel like you have to add it to yours). It's chic, slimming, and pairs well with almost any other colour.

White: Clean, fresh, and timeless, white is a favourite for its simplicity and ability to create a crisp and sophisticated look (again, don't feel like you have to add it to yours).

Navy Blue: A sophisticated alternative to black, navy blue is a popular colour for both formal and casual wear.

Grey: A neutral and elegant choice, various shades of grey can complement many other colours in an outfit.

Blush Pink: Soft and feminine, blush pink has become a beloved colour in fashion, particularly for spring and summer looks.

Burgundy: This rich, deep red colour is a popular choice for fall and winter, adding warmth and sophistication to outfits.

Olive Green: A versatile and earthy hue, olive green works well with many other colours and is a great choice for casual wear.

Mustard Yellow: A trendy and vibrant colour, mustard yellow has gained popularity in recent years for its bold and warm appeal.

Royal Blue: A bold and regal shade, royal blue makes a statement and works well for both daytime and evening looks.

Emerald Green: This jewel tone exudes elegance and is a popular choice for special occasions and evening wear.

Red: A bold and attention-grabbing colour, red is often associated with confidence and power.

Pastel Blue: Soft and soothing, pastel blue is a favourite for creating calm and fresh looks.

Camel: A warm and sophisticated neutral, camel adds a touch of luxury to outfits.

This can be a great choice for a bag.

Lavender: A soft and romantic colour, lavender is favoured for its dreamy and feminine appeal. This colour is perfect for spring.

Teal: This vibrant blue-green hue is a striking choice that works well in both casual and formal settings.

5. Style icons - *Style icons could include any prominent celebrities, fashion designers, models, musicians, influencers, and other public figures who inspire you and your style. Whose fashion is inspiring you right now? It may be worth creating a mood board on Pinterest, or even a collection on Instagram.*

Writing down these answers will provide you with a basic understanding of your personal style. The following task will allow you to further develop this understanding.

Activity 2

It is time to get creative. Start with a 1-2-week period during which you take photos of your outfits daily—this may sound excessive, but it will be worth it! These can just be simple mirror selfies; they don't need to be overproduced. Style is a highly visual medium, and these pictures can provide valuable insights. Over the two-week period, add these photos to a folder on your phone so they are all in one place. Once you have gathered all your photos over this time period, reflect and answer the following questions:

- Which are your favourite outfits, and why? How did wearing this outfit make you feel?
- What are your least favourite outfits, and why? How did it make you feel when you wore it?

- Try to describe your style in a few words based on the outfits you liked.
- Take note of the most frequently worn pieces, colours, styles, and silhouettes throughout the period. What did you feel most comfortable and confident in?
- Assess how easy or challenging it was for you to select the outfits each morning.
- Analyse the messages that your current appearance might be conveying to others.

You can also spend a couple of hours going through your wardrobe, putting together some outfits, and answering the questions above. Writing down these answers will really allow you to see what you do and don't like in your wardrobe currently, and you can adapt your wardrobe from here.

Activity 3

The Three Word Method is a fun and innovative styling tool that aims to define and capture your own unique personal style through just three carefully chosen descriptive words. Everyone will have a different outcome from this task. You can refer to these words in the future when thinking about your personal. The concept of using language to delve into your fashion identity caught many people's attention on TikTok in 2022. The now-famous TikTok influencer, Allison Bornstein, developed the method with clear intention. The Three Word Method involves selecting three adjectives that encapsulate your personal style or the style you aspire to embody. This task really is proof that not every TikTok trend is a fad.

While the basic idea of choosing three descriptive words might sound easy, it may take a brainstorming session, and then you can revisit the list and refine these words over time. By thoughtfully considering and combining three words that truly resonate with your fashion preferences, you can gain valuable insights into your personal style identity. Whether you lean towards classic, bohemian, edgy, chic, or any other style, the Three Word Method empowers you to articulate and define your fashion choices in a concise yet meaningful way. This approach can serve as a guiding light in curating a wardrobe that authentically reflects who you are and how you want to present yourself to the world.

If you need more inspiration on what words to use or where to start with this task, visit Allison Bernstein's TikTok account.

Below are 50 words that you can start using to explore The Three Word Method:

- Classic
- Bohemian
- Edgy
- Chic
- Romantic
- Casual
- Vintage
- Sophisticated
- Retro
- Minimalist
- Artsy
- Glamorous
- Eclectic
- Preppy
- Sporty
- Urban
- Elegant
- Grunge
- Effortless
- Trendy

- Whimsical
- Rocker
- Feminine
- Modern
- Bold
- Casual
- Colourful
- Classy
- Nautical
- Timeless
- Masculine
- Boho-chic
- Streetwear
- Tailored
- Experimental
- Quirky
- Retro-modern
- Laid-back
- Dramatic
- Ethereal
- Utilitarian
- Statement
- Rustic
- Monochromatic
- Sustainable
- Dapper
- Asymmetric
- Playful
- Artsy
- Vintage-inspired

Tip: If you are stuck on what words you could use, you can ask your friends and family to describe your style and use these words as a starting point.

Once you have identified your words using the Three Word Method, you can refer to them at any time in the future when you look to introduce something new to your wardrobe or you go to clear out your closet.

3

Editing Your Current Wardrobe

Before we expand and add to your wardrobe, it is important to sort through what you currently have in your closet and see what you are working with. It is most likely that you have not worn 50% of your wardrobe in the past year. Clearing out your wardrobe is a great way to declutter and make space for more curated and fashionable pieces to add to your wardrobe (we will get to that later). To effectively clear out your wardrobe, set aside dedicated time when you can focus solely on this task. This may sound boring, but trust me, it will be worth it when you are looking 10/10 in your restyled wardrobe. Set aside an afternoon or an hour in the evening after work across a week so you have enough time to thoroughly assess each item and make thoughtful decisions on what will stay and what will go. Of course, you can make this task more exciting by listening to your favourite album or putting on your favourite podcast.

Take one item out of your wardrobe at a time, then decide if the item should stay or go with the following techniques. Taking everything out at once and then sorting through everything can make this process overwhelming. Slow and steady wins the race! Don't feel as though you have to sort this out in one shift.

Divide your clothing into various categories, such as tops, bottoms, shoes, dresses, outerwear, and accessories. This sorting process helps you see the quantity and variety of items you have in each category. This will also allow you to tackle one clothing category at a time. Create separate piles for items you want to keep, donate or sell, and items that need further consideration. As you go through each item, be really honest with yourself about whether you still wear and enjoy it. Do you have multiple black tops? Do you need both? Consider factors like fit, condition, and how frequently you ACTUALLY wear each piece. Ask yourself if it aligns with your current style, if it makes you feel confident, and if it serves a purpose in your wardrobe. For example, you may not wear your ski suit every day, but it still has a purpose.

Quality over quantity is really true when it comes to your wardrobe. When curating your wardrobe, focus on quality pieces that are well-made and durable. Investing in higher-quality items means they'll last longer, which reduces the need for frequent replacements, and you will ultimately save money in the long term too. It is a double win!

Applying the famous KonMari Method can also be helpful to figure out what you really want to keep in your wardrobe. Use Marie Kondo's "spark joy" method to determine which items to keep and which need to go. If an item brings you joy and makes you feel good when you wear it, it's worth keeping. If it no longer sparks joy, it's time to say goodbye. Additionally, evaluate if certain items are outdated or overly trendy. While it's good to embrace trends, prioritise timeless pieces that have longevity and can be styled in multiple ways. If you like the idea of this method, it is worth checking out Marie Kondo's book 'The Life Changing Magic of Tidying' which will help you organise your entire home, not just your closet.

Make sure to check for fit and condition. Ensure that each item fits well and flatters your body shape. Let go of items that no longer fit or that require extensive alterations. Assess the condition of each piece and discard items that are damaged, stained, or worn beyond repair. Items that are in good condition but no longer serve you can be donated to charitable organisations or sold through platforms like consignment stores, Ebay, Depop, or Vinted.

Once you've cleared out unwanted items, reorganise your wardrobe in a way that makes the remaining pieces easily visible and accessible. Your wardrobe should be a beautiful and organised place that makes you feel happy. Consider using organising tools like hangers, dividers, or storage boxes to maintain order. Building a versatile capsule wardrobe consisting of essential and interchangeable pieces is also a great approach. This allows for easier outfit creation and ensures that your remaining items are fashionable and wearable in various combinations.

Going forward, adopt a more intentional and mindful approach to shopping while considering tasks 1, 2 & 3 that you have already completed. Before making a new purchase, consider if the item aligns with your personal style, fits your wardrobe needs, and can be worn multiple ways. Always refer back to the words you chose during the Three Word Method. Avoid impulse buying an item just because it is on sale or you have seen a random trend explode. Think about whether that trend is really for you. By following these techniques, you can clear out your wardrobe and create a fashionable and curated collection that reflects your personal style and brings you joy when getting dressed.

As your style evolves, continue to declutter your wardrobe periodically. This will help you maintain a curated collection that truly represents your personal style. Remember that finding your personal style is a journey, and it's essential to enjoy the process. Take your time to explore different options and choose pieces that make you feel confident and comfortable. Every 6 months or so, you can run yourself through tasks 1,2 & 3 to ensure your personal style is adapting and evolving as you grow in your life. It is okay for your favourite style icons to change or to eventually hate a piece in your wardrobe that you once loved. Your wardrobe should be a reflection of your individuality and make you excited about getting dressed every day.

When placing items back into your wardrobe, doing so aesthetically not only creates a visually appealing space but also makes it easier to find and coordinate outfits. A well-organised wardrobe can be a source of inspiration and enjoyment every time you get dressed in the morning. Here are some stunning tips to help you organise your wardrobe aesthetically:

Colour Coordination: Arrange your clothes within each category by colour, creating a visually pleasing gradient. You can organise from light to dark shades or group similar colours together. Colour-coordinating your wardrobe makes it easier to spot pieces and can be aesthetically pleasing. The psychological impact of colours enhances the overall appeal, evoking positive emotions when getting dressed. The versatility of such wardrobes allows for effortless mixing and matching, offering a wide range of outfit possibilities.

Matching Hangers: Invest in sleek uniform hangers to create a neat and cohesive appearance. Velvet or wooden hangers are excellent choices, as they add a touch of elegance and prevent clothes from slipping off. Go for hangers that suit your personal style and aesthetic.

Open Shelving: If your wardrobe allows it, consider incorporating open shelves or display units. Use these shelves to showcase your favourite accessories, shoes, or handbags, adding a personalised and decorative touch to the space. This can be great to use on your statement bags or as an ornament in your room.

Drawer Organisers: Keep smaller items like socks, underwear, scarves, and belts organised using drawer dividers or organisers. No one wants to see these pieces! This prevents all the clutter and ensures that everything has its designated place. If it doesn't have a home, then you should expect a messy wardrobe to happen at some point.

Off-Season Items: If your wardrobe is limited in space, store off-season clothes in under-bed storage containers or in a separate closet. You could even use a spare suitcase! This keeps your main wardrobe area focused on current-season items, making it easier to navigate. You can schedule a seasonal wardrobe changeover to do the big swap! This can also be a great time to further organise your wardrobe.

Fold and Stack Items: For items like jeans, sweaters, and t-shirts, fold them neatly and stack them vertically in drawers or on shelves. This technique saves space and allows you to see all your options at a glance. Folding is such an underrated basic skill, but this is definitely worth learning how to do properly from a Youtube tutorial.

Statement Pieces: Hang statement pieces, such as dresses or statement jackets, in a prominent spot within your wardrobe. Not only will they be well preserved, but they'll also serve as a source of fashion inspiration when planning outfits. If you have an investment bag that you love the look of, don't be afraid to display it on a shelf in a room. Accessories don't just need to be for your outfits; they can also take your interiors to the next level.

By applying these tips, you can create an aesthetically pleasing and well-organised wardrobe that not only makes getting dressed easier and more enjoyable but also serves as a reflection of your personal style and attention to detail. A visually appealing wardrobe space can positively impact your fashion choices and inspire you to explore new outfit combinations every morning.

Once your wardrobe is organised, you need to keep it like this. The success of a wonderful wardrobe lies in its maintenance and adaptability. You need to ensure that your wardrobe remains functional and fashionable over time. Sometimes this is easier said than done, so consider the following maintenance steps:

The Hanger Technique: Turn all your hangers backward at the beginning of the season or after your wardrobe is tidied up. As you wear an item, hang it back in the closet with the hanger facing the usual direction. After a few months, you'll easily identify which clothes you haven't worn. Consider letting go of those items that have been untouched. This will allow you to continue to define your wardrobe.

Set Aside Dedicated Time: Allocate a specific time in your calendar when you can focus solely on decluttering your wardrobe. This ensures that you have enough time to thoroughly assess each item and make thoughtful decisions. Add a diary reminder at the end of each month for regular maintenance. Your wardrobe should be a place of joy and happiness, so you need to ensure you review it, just like you would with your skincare routine, if something is not working for you.

Seasonal Refresh: With the changing seasons, review your capsule wardrobe and adjust the pieces to suit the weather, occasions in your life, and your evolving style preferences.

Tailoring and Repairs: Repair or tailor any damaged items to extend their lifespan and ensure a perfect fit. If you have clothes that you love but rarely wear due to minor issues like loose hems or outdated styles, consider repurposing or up-cycling them. You can turn a long dress into a stylish top or spice it up by adding patches or embroidery to update a jacket. Sometimes you don't need to get rid of everything you don't want.

Mindful Additions: Be thoughtful when adding new pieces to your wardrobe. Ensure that they align with your existing style and can be easily integrated into your outfits. As your wardrobe evolves, continue to prioritise quality and versatility over impulse buying. When buying something new, try to visualise three different outfits that you could wear the piece with from your current wardrobe.

Activity 4

The wardrobe clean-out and reorganisation! It is time to put what you have just learned into action and whittle down your wardrobe. Take it step by step! Firstly, clear out what you do and don't want to keep. Then reorganise your wardrobe. Finally, taking steps to ensure your wardrobe remains up-to-date with your personal style.

4

Building a Capsule Wardrobe

Combining a capsule wardrobe with your personal style is like creating a fashion masterpiece that reflects the true essence of who you are within your wardrobe. It's about curating a collection of clothing that not only simplifies your daily choices but also showcases your unique taste and personality. So, let's dive into the art of blending these two elements seamlessly.

First and foremost, embrace the core principles of a capsule wardrobe. Think of it as the backbone of your style canvas, the blank slate upon which you'll paint your sartorial dreams. Carefully select timeless and versatile pieces that form the foundation of your wardrobe. Classic items like well-fitted jeans, a tailored blazer, a crisp white shirt, and maybe a little black dress are the building blocks that will complement any personal style. However, it is important to remember that not everyone's capsule wardrobe pieces will look the same.

At its core, a capsule wardrobe emphasises quality over quantity. With the goal of owning a carefully curated selection of clothes, typically consisting of 30 to 50 items, including clothing, shoes, and accessories. These items should be versatile, durable, and suited to your lifestyle, allowing you to create a wide range of outfits while reducing fashion fatigue and wardrobe clutter.

A capsule wardrobe operates on five fundamental principles that form its backbone. Firstly, versatility ensures each item can effortlessly team up with multiple others, which can help multiply outfit possibilities. Secondly, the timelessness factor takes centre stage when thinking about a capsule wardrobe, favouring classic wardrobe staples that defy the fleeting grasp of seasonal trends. However, this doesn't mean you need to opt for boring pieces because they will be timeless. Thirdly, quality is a must; only the finest, well-crafted garments from durable materials should earn a spot in your wardrobe lineup. Fourthly, a colour scheme that matches your personal style should be considered. While adhering to the principles of a capsule wardrobe, it's essential to preserve and express your unique personal style. Your wardrobe should reflect your tastes, preferences, and lifestyle.

A well-organised capsule wardrobe should be prepared to tackle the ever-changing seasons, ensuring you have suitable attire for various weather conditions. To achieve this, consider dividing your wardrobe into seasonal capsules for spring/summer and autumn/winter, allowing you to rotate and store items accordingly. Embrace the power of layering by investing in versatile pieces like cardigans, lightweight jackets, and scarves, which can be effortlessly added or removed based on the weather's whims. Additionally, opt for multi-seasonal items that gracefully transition across different seasons with the right layering or creative styling, adding flexibility and longevity to your curated collection. With this thoughtful approach to seasonal planning, your capsule wardrobe will be perfect to see you through the year, ready to adapt and shine in any weather.

There are many benefits to building a capsule wardrobe that go beyond just fashion. Firstly, it simplifies decision-making when it comes to getting dressed in the morning. With a few pieces that should complement one another, you spend less time deciding what to wear each day, streamlining your morning routine. You also save time and money as a capsule wardrobe encourages mindful purchasing, preventing impulse buys and unnecessary expenses on clothes you will ultimately rarely wear. By reducing clutter and becoming more sustainable by investing in high-quality, long-lasting pieces and reducing clothing consumption, you contribute to a more eco-friendly approach to fashion. A capsule wardrobe tends to be particularly convenient for travel, as it allows you to pack light while still having enough outfit options.

Activity 5

Once you have a clear understanding of your personal style as well as the fundamentals of a capsule wardrobe, it's time to define the essential pieces that will form the foundation of your capsule wardrobe. Below is a list of some key categories you may want to include in your capsule wardrobe. Start to compile a list of the pieces you want and that you already have. Once you have your want list, you do not need to do a bulk buy of all of these pieces in one go. You can consider adding a few items to your wardrobe each month. Remember to do your research on these items to ensure they are of good quality and that they suit your personal style by revisiting tasks 1,2 & 3.

Classic Basics: Start with classic basics that are timeless and versatile. These include well-fitting jeans, tailored trousers, a white button-down shirt, a neutral blazer, and a little black dress for any occasion. A neutral-coloured sweater in a cosy fabric is perfect for colder months. It can be layered with shirts or blouses or worn on its own with jeans or trousers, ensuring both warmth and style. A well-fitted white t-shirt is a wardrobe essential that provides the perfect base for layering or as a standalone piece. It can be paired with jeans, skirts, shorts, or under blazers, offering endless outfit possibilities.

Tops and Blouses: Choose a mix of tops and blouses in different colours and styles that can be easily layered and paired with different kinds of bottoms, from jeans to skirts. A crisp and well-fitted white shirt is a timeless staple that can be dressed up for formal occasions or dressed down for a casual, chic look. It pairs beautifully with jeans, skirts, trousers, or layered under blazers, making it a versatile and indispensable piece.

Bottoms: Invest in bottoms that suit your lifestyle, such as skirts, shorts, and pants in coordinating colours. This can include different styles of denim jeans or different styles of skirts. A high-quality pair of jeans in a classic wash is a must-have for any capsule wardrobe. Opt for a style that flatters your body shape and complements your personal style. Jeans are incredibly versatile and can be worn with various tops and shoes, making them a go-to item for everyday outfits. A midi skirt in a flattering silhouette and neutral colour can be dressed up or down for various occasions. It pairs well with blouses, sweaters, or t-shirts, making it a versatile and feminine addition to your capsule wardrobe.

Dresses: Include dresses that can be dressed up or down for various occasions. Consider the different occasions you may wear these dresses to and how you would style them for each occasion. The iconic little black dress is a timeless piece that exudes elegance and sophistication. Choose a style that suits your body shape and can be dressed up or down with accessories. The LBD is perfect for formal events, parties, or even a night out with friends.

Tailored Pieces: A well-tailored blazer instantly elevates any outfit and adds a polished touch to your look. It can be worn with jeans for a smart-casual vibe or paired with trousers or a skirt for a more professional setting. Choose a neutral colour like black, navy, or grey to ensure easy coordination with other pieces. A pair of well-tailored trousers in a classic cut and neutral colour are essential for a polished and professional look. These trousers can be dressed up with a blouse and heels for work or dressed down with a t-shirt and sneakers for a more relaxed style.

Outerwear: Select outerwear pieces such as a tailored coat, a leather jacket, or a fur coat that complement your style. A classic trench coat is not only stylish but also practical, offering protection from the elements while adding sophistication to your outfit. Opt for a neutral colour like beige or khaki, as it complements a wide range of outfits and works well in both formal and casual settings. Think about what can be worn in different seasons; for example, a cardigan might be better for the warmer months.

Shoes: Opt for versatile shoes that are comfortable and suitable for different occasions, such as a pair of flats, heels, or sneakers. Invest in a pair of comfortable flats that can be worn all day without sacrificing style. Whether it's ballet flats, loafers, or pointed-toe flats, they add a touch of elegance to your outfits while ensuring comfort and practicality. Versatile ankle boots are a staple for any cold-weather wardrobe. They can be paired with dresses, skirts, or jeans, adding a touch of edge and sophistication to your outfits.

Accessories: Complete your capsule wardrobe with accessories like bags, sunglasses, belts, and jewellery that can elevate and personalise your outfits.

These key pieces will serve as the building blocks of your capsule wardrobe, providing you with endless possibilities for creating stylish and cohesive outfits for any occasion. With these essentials at your disposal, you'll find that dressing up becomes more effortless and enjoyable, while also embracing a more sustainable and mindful approach to fashion.

Now comes the exciting part—infusing your capsule wardrobe with your personal flair. This is where you get to add the pops of colour, textures, and patterns that make your heart skip a beat. Take a look at your current wardrobe and identify the clothing that truly resonates with you. Maybe you're drawn to bohemian maxi dresses, bold geometric prints, or vintage-inspired accessories. Embrace these elements like a painter embracing their favourite hues and incorporate them into your capsule collection.

Don't shy away from experimenting and mixing styles. Try pairing your edgy leather jacket with a flowy floral dress, or match your tailored blazer with distressed denim. The key is to let your creativity soar and break traditional fashion rules with confidence. You will have a combo you love.

Activity 6

A well-defined colour palette is a key element of a cohesive and functional capsule wardrobe. By selecting a limited range of colours that complement each other, you can easily mix and match pieces to create various outfits. Consider the following categories and take notes on them:

Skin tone: Determining your skin's undertone is crucial. It can be warm, cool, or neutral. A simple trick is to observe the veins on your wrist. If they appear green, you likely have warm undertones; if they look blue or purple, you probably have cool undertones. If you can't quite tell, you might have a neutral undertone, which means you can wear a wide range of colours.

Neutral Base: Start with a foundation of neutral colours, such as black, white, grey, navy, and beige. These versatile shades form the base of your wardrobe and can be easily paired with bolder colours. What neutrals are missing from your wardrobe? Is there a reason you haven't included them in your wardrobe yet?

Accent Colours: Introduce a few accent colours that complement your neutral base. These can be shades that reflect your personal style or colours that you feel confident wearing. What colours do you feel best in?

Cohesive Palette: Ensure that all the colours in your capsule wardrobe work harmoniously together. This cohesiveness allows for effortless outfit creation and coordination. Do you enjoy bright colours, pastels, or maybe darker shades?

Tip: Take time to play dress-up in front of a well-lit mirror. Hold different coloured fabrics or papers close to your face and observe how they affect your complexion. Colours that make you look radiant and awake are strong contenders for your palette.

Activity 7

While the primary focus of a capsule wardrobe is on timeless and versatile pieces, adding a few statement pieces can elevate your outfits and add personality to your style. Consider each of the below categories and write down three pieces that you have or want to add to your wardrobe.

Statement Accessories: Incorporate bold and eye-catching accessories, such as a colourful scarf, a statement necklace, or a unique handbag. Accessories are the secret weapon to elevate your style game even further. Just as a sculptor adds intricate details to their masterpiece, accessorise thoughtfully to enhance your outfits. Statement jewellery, scarves, hats, or even a killer pair of shoes can instantly transform a simple look into a bold fashion statement that represents your unique taste.

Trendy Items: Introduce a few trendy pieces that align with your personal style and can be incorporated into your capsule wardrobe without over-whelming the overall aesthetic.

Signature Pieces: Consider including one or two signature pieces that reflect your individuality and are a true representation of your personal style.

As you refine your capsule wardrobe, stay true to yourself and your lifestyle.

Like a novelist crafting a character, think about the story you want your wardrobe to tell. Consider the occasions you frequently encounter, whether it's for work, casual outings, or special events, and ensure your capsule pieces cater to those needs. Don't forget comfort, functionality, and versatility; these elements will ensure your capsule wardrobe stays practical and enjoyable. We will cover this in greater detail later!

Allow your style to evolve and adapt over time. Just as an artist's style evolves with each masterpiece, your fashion sense will naturally grow and change. Embrace the journey and be open to discovering new styles and trends. Remember, your capsule wardrobe is a reflection of you, and it should evolve as you do.

Building a capsule wardrobe is a transformative and empowering process that promotes simplicity, sustainability, and self-awareness. By understanding your personal style, defining a cohesive colour palette, and curating a collection of versatile and timeless pieces, you can create a wardrobe that aligns with your lifestyle, enhances your self-confidence, and brings joy to your daily dressing routine. Combining a capsule wardrobe with personal style is about creating a harmonious blend of classic, versatile pieces with unique, expressive elements that make you stand out. So, embrace your creativity and let your capsule wardrobe be the ultimate expression of your fabulous, one-of-a-kind self!

5

Trendy & True To You

Following fashion trends can have its drawbacks and might not always be the best approach to building a personal style. Here are some reasons why blindly adhering to fashion trends can be seen as negative.

One of the main downsides of following fashion trends is the potential loss of individuality. When everyone is wearing the same trendy pieces, it can be challenging to stand out and express your unique personality through your style. Your fashion choices might end up feeling more like a clone of what's popular than a reflection of who you truly are.

Fashion trends change rapidly, with new styles emerging each season. Following trends can lead to constant shopping and a "buy and discard" culture, which can be detrimental to the environment and contribute to excessive consumerism. This fast-paced consumption can also strain personal finances and lead to a wardrobe full of items that quickly go out of style.

Fashion trends are often heavily influenced by mass media, celebrities, and influencers. While these influences can introduce exciting new styles, they can also promote unrealistic beauty standards and create pressure to conform to certain looks. This can negatively impact self-esteem and body image, as individuals may feel inadequate if they don't match the perceived "ideal" portrayed in the media.

Following trends may prioritise quantity over quality. Fast fashion retailers, in particular, often produce inexpensive and trendy clothing, but the quality might be compromised. These items might not last long, leading to more waste and a higher demand for new trends.

Relying solely on fashion trends may limit your creative expression and prevent you from exploring different styles that truly resonate with you. Personal style is an opportunity for self-expression and should be a reflection of your unique tastes and interests rather than conforming to fleeting trends.

Keeping up with every new trend can be financially taxing. Trendy items are often priced higher due to their popularity, leading to a constant need to spend to stay "on trend." This can strain budgets and create a sense of financial insecurity.

Fashion trends come and go quickly, and the excitement of owning the latest "it" piece can fade just as fast. The euphoria of being in style may be short-lived, leaving you in constant pursuit of the next big trend for temporary gratification.

While exploring fashion trends can be fun and add a fresh touch to your wardrobe, blindly following them can have negative consequences. It's important to strike a balance and use trends as inspiration while staying true to your individuality and values. Focusing on building a timeless and versatile wardrobe with pieces that truly resonate with you allows for a more sustainable and authentic approach to personal style. Staying on trend while staying true to our personal style is like a fashion tug of war, but fear not, for it can be done!

Firstly, it's essential to be selective when incorporating trend-forward pieces into your wardrobe. Stay informed about current fashion trends, but choose those that truly resonate with your personal style. Integrate trendy items that align with your aesthetic and can seamlessly complement your existing wardrobe. This way, you'll feel confident and authentic while embracing what's new and exciting in the fashion world.

Don't be afraid to put your own spin on the trends you love. Take inspiration from the latest runway looks or street style icons, but adapt them to suit your unique taste. Mix and match classic pieces from your wardrobe to create ensembles that express your individuality while staying current.

Pay attention to the colours and patterns that are popular in each season. You can incorporate trendy colours or prints into your outfits through accessories like scarves, shoes, or bags. This allows you to experiment with the latest trends without committing to a full wardrobe overhaul.

Focus on the details. Small touches like statement jewellery, bold belts, or unique eyewear can instantly elevate your look and keep it fresh without compromising your personal style. Accessories offer a fantastic opportunity to play with trends in a way that feels authentic to you.

Don't forget to consider your lifestyle when embracing trends. While some styles may look stunning on the runway, they might not be practical for your daily activities. Choose trends that align with your routine, making it easier to incorporate them seamlessly into your wardrobe.

Remember that fashion is ever-evolving, and it's okay to experiment and evolve with it. Embrace the opportunity to try new things and step out of your comfort zone. Allow your style to adapt and grow while staying true to the essence of who you are. Staying on trend while maintaining your personal style is about finding a harmonious blend of what's current and what's authentic to you. Be selective, put your own spin on trends, play with colours and patterns, and embrace experimentation. With these tips, you'll confidently conquer the fashion tightrope and emerge as a true style maven.

Activity 8

Next time you consider adding a trend to your wardrobe, ask yourself, 'Would I wear this if it wasn't actually a trend?'. While trends can introduce us to new fashion possibilities, we should avoid blindly following them just because they're popular. Take a moment to assess whether you genuinely like the pieces and would wear them regardless of their trend status. Be honest with yourself! If the answer is yes, then go for it! If you are still unsure, wait a week or so and ask yourself the same question. If you are still not sure if you should go ahead with the trend, it is probably best to leave it.

6

Fashion Influences

Personal style can be influenced by a wide range of factors, which can play a key role in shaping someone's fashion preferences and choices. Understanding what can influence your style is crucial because it empowers you to make informed decisions.

One of the influences on personal style is an individual's personality. Introverted individuals may prefer more subdued and understated styles, while extroverted individuals may gravitate towards bold and expressive clothing choices. Our personality traits often dictate the colours, patterns, and silhouettes that make us feel most comfortable and confident, resulting in a unique and authentic personal style. This isn't always an accurate rule, but it's a pattern you may see frequently.

Cultural influences play a vital role in shaping personal style. Our cultural background and heritage can impact the way we dress, incorporating traditional elements and garments into our modern fashion choices. Cultural influences can be seen in the use of specific fabrics, colours, accessories, and even certain garment styles that carry a sense of identity and pride.

The way we dress is often influenced by our lifestyle and occupation, too. For instance, individuals with active lifestyles may prefer comfortable and practical clothing, while those in more formal professions might opt for tailored and professional attire. Lifestyle choices, such as hobbies and activities, can also influence personal style, with some individuals embracing sporty or casual looks while others prefer more artistic or bohemian styles.

Our personal values and beliefs can be reflected in our fashion choices. Ethical and sustainable fashion have become increasingly important to many individuals, leading them to opt for eco-friendly and ethically produced clothing. Some may choose to wear clothing that supports causes or expresses their beliefs, using fashion as a means of advocating for social and environmental issues.

Personal style is often influenced by an individual's body shape and proportions. Understanding your body type can lead to clothing choices that enhance and flatter specific features, resulting in a more confident and comfortable appearance. People may gravitate towards certain cuts and styles that accentuate their best attributes and create a balanced silhouette. We will discuss a whole lot more about your body shape and clothing fit in the coming chapters.

Peer groups and social circles can also influence personal style. People may be inspired or influenced by the fashion choices of friends, family members, or influencers within their community. The desire to fit in or stand out within a particular social context can impact the way individuals dress and present themselves.

The fashion industry and media significantly influence personal style by showcasing the latest trends and styles. Fashion magazines, social media, runway shows, and celebrity fashion often lead people to incorporate current trends into their wardrobes. Social media has had a profound influence on personal style, revolutionising the way people discover, express, and shape their fashion preferences. The impact of platforms like Instagram, Pinterest, and TikTok has made fashion trends and styles more accessible than ever before.

Social media exposes us all to a wide range of fashion trends from around the world. Influencers, bloggers, and celebrities showcase their unique styles, introducing users to new and diverse fashion choices. This exposure helps individuals explore different looks and incorporate elements they resonate with into their own personal style. It's also important to give credit to these platforms, as they act as a treasure trove of fashion inspiration. Users can discover new brands, designers, and fashion ideas that they might not have encountered otherwise. This continuous stream of inspiration fuels creativity and encourages people to experiment with their clothing choices. Influencers on social media platforms play a significant role in shaping personal style trends. People often look up to influencers as fashion authorities, leading to the emulation of their style choices. However, it's essential for individuals to balance this influence with their own unique preferences and not feel pressured to copy trends that don't align with their identity. Social media creates a sense of community around fashion and personal style. Users can connect with like-minded individuals who share their fashion interests and engage in conversations about trends, brands, and styling tips. This sense of community fosters a supportive environment for self-expression through fashion. In addition, social media platforms provide real-time updates on fashion events, runway shows, and new collections. This immediacy allows followers to stay informed about the latest trends and be at the forefront of fashion discussions. Social media has also encouraged a surge in do-it-yourself (DIY) fashion and up-cycling projects. Users share tutorials and ideas for revamping old clothing or creating unique pieces, promoting sustainability, and reducing waste.

Personal style is shaped by a multitude of influences, ranging from individual personality traits and cultural background to fashion trends, media, and lifestyle choices. Additionally, personal values, body shape, and peer influences all play a significant role in defining and evolving an individual's fashion preferences. The combination of these factors contributes to the rich diversity of personal styles seen across the world, each one reflecting the unique essence and identity of the individual who embraces it. However, it is essential to acknowledge that there can be potential negatives associated with the influence of fashion on individuals and society.

Fashion trends and societal expectations can create pressure to conform to certain styles or ideals. Individuals may feel compelled to follow the latest trends, even if those styles don't resonate with their personal preferences or values. This pressure to conform can lead to a loss of individuality and result in people sacrificing their unique sense of style to fit in with the crowd.

Fashion's emphasis on certain body types and beauty standards can negatively affect body image and self-esteem. The industry's portrayal of unrealistic body ideals may lead to feelings of inadequacy and a distorted perception of your own body. This pressure to conform to a particular aesthetic can foster body dissatisfaction and contribute to the development of eating disorders and other mental health issues.

The influence of fashion can foster a culture of materialism and consumerism where the focus is placed on acquiring the latest clothing and accessories rather than valuing inner qualities and personal growth. Constantly chasing new trends can lead to excessive consumption and wastefulness, contributing to environmental issues such as fast fashion's impact on the planet. The fashion industry is known for its significant environmental impact, from water usage and pollution to the production of clothing materials. Constantly changing fashion trends and fast-fashion practises contribute to a cycle of waste as clothing is discarded and replaced with new pieces at a rapid pace. This has serious consequences for the environment and sustainability.

The pursuit of personal style and fashion trends can be financially taxing, especially when people feel compelled to constantly update their wardrobe to keep up with the latest looks. For some, this may lead to overspending, debt, or financial strain as fashion becomes a significant expense in their lives.

Despite its positive aspects, social media can also foster pressure and comparison when it comes to personal style. Constant exposure to curated images of seemingly perfect fashion can lead to feelings of inadequacy or a desire to conform to unrealistic beauty standards. It's crucial for individuals to approach social media with discernment, maintaining a balance between being inspired by others and staying true to their authentic selves. By using social media mindfully, you can harness its potential for a positive impact on your personal style and self-expression.

While personal style can be an empowering form of self-expression, it is essential to recognise and address the potential negatives associated with fashion influence. The pressure to conform, materialism, body image issues, financial strain, exclusion, environmental impact, and distraction from inner growth are all aspects that individuals and society should be mindful of when engaging with the world of fashion. Striking a balance between embracing personal style and maintaining self-awareness and critical thinking is crucial to fostering a healthy and holistic relationship with fashion.

There are some things to consider to avoid being overly influenced by fashion and to maintain a healthy relationship with your personal style that you have established. It's important to cultivate self-awareness and understand your values, interests, and personal preferences. Being in touch with your authentic self will help you make conscious fashion choices that align with who you are, rather than being solely influenced by external trends. Experiment with different looks and try to identify what makes you feel confident and comfortable. Develop a signature style that reflects your personality and individuality, regardless of whether it aligns with current fashion trends. Take yourself back to tasks 1, 2 & 3 to ensure your personal style is staying authentic.

Be mindful of your shopping habits and avoid impulsive purchases driven solely by fashion trends. Before buying new clothing, consider whether the item complements your existing wardrobe and if it's something you genuinely need and will wear frequently. Focus on quality pieces that are versatile and well-made rather than accumulating a large quantity of cheap and low-quality fast-fashion items. Investing in timeless, durable pieces not only benefits the environment but also ensures your wardrobe remains relevant beyond fleeting trends. Resist the urge to compare yourself to others based on appearance or fashion choices. Embrace your unique style, and remember that fashion is subjective and personal. Celebrate the diversity of individuality in style, including your own. Reject unrealistic beauty standards perpetuated by the fashion industry and celebrate your body as it is.

Take ownership of yourself to learn about the ethical and environmental impact of the fashion industry. Understanding the consequences of fast fashion and unsustainable practises can influence your purchasing decisions and encourage you to support more sustainable and ethical brands. While personal style is enjoyable and expressive, remember that it is just one facet of your identity. Focus on developing inner qualities, skills, and passions that define you beyond your appearance.

Reduce your exposure to fashion media and advertising if you find that it negatively impacts your self-esteem or leads to excessive materialism. Curate your social media feeds to follow accounts that show you the fashion you love. And don't forget, you can hit the unfollow button at any time.

Surround yourself with friends and family who appreciate you for who you are, regardless of your fashion choices. Having a supportive network can boost your self-confidence and reinforce the importance of staying true to yourself. Staying true to yourself and avoiding excessive influences from the fashion world involve cultivating self-awareness, defining your personal style, and mindful consumption. By making conscious choices and focusing on what truly matters, you can create a balanced and empowered relationship with your personal style.

7

Work & Event Dressing

At times, it can be really difficult to find your personal style when you are at work or have to dress within the rules. Dressing in your personal style during your personal time is often much easier for several reasons. Firstly, outside of formal work settings, there are generally no dress codes or strict guidelines to adhere to. This lack of restrictions allows you the freedom to express yourself through your clothing choices without the pressure to conform to a particular image or standard.

Secondly, during your personal time, you are in a more relaxed and casual environment. Whether you're spending time with friends, engaging in hobbies, or simply enjoying leisure activities, the atmosphere is often laid-back and informal. This relaxed setting fosters a sense of comfort and ease, making it easier to dress in a way that reflects your personality and preferences.

Additionally, personal time is an opportunity for self-expression and individuality. It's a chance to step away from the demands of the professional world and embrace your true self. Dressing in your personal style allows you to communicate who you are, what you love, and what makes you unique without the need to conform to societal or workplace norms. Dressing in your personal style during your personal time is a way to connect with others who share similar interests or aesthetics. Fashion choices can be like a language that communicates your passions and values, helping you find like-minded individuals and fostering a sense of belonging. The absence of time constraints and the focus on personal enjoyment contribute to the ease of dressing in your personal style during your personal time. Unlike the rushed mornings before work, you have the luxury of taking your time, trying out different outfits, and truly enjoying the process of getting dressed.

Dressing in your personal style during your personal time is easier due to the lack of dress codes, the relaxed and casual setting, the opportunity for self-expression, and the absence of time pressure. It's a liberating and enjoyable experience that allows you to embrace your individuality and showcase your unique fashion choices to the world. In addition to this, personal style can be challenging to maintain at work for several reasons. Firstly, many workplaces have strict dress codes that dictate what employees can and cannot wear. These guidelines are often put in place to maintain a certain level of professionalism and consistency within the organisation. While they serve a purpose, they can limit individual self-expression and make it difficult to showcase personal style.

The fear of judgement can discourage individuals from expressing their personal style at work. They might worry that their fashion choices could be perceived as unprofessional or distracting, leading them to opt for safer, more conservative options. Striking a balance between style and professionalism becomes an internal struggle, making it hard to confidently embrace one's unique fashion choices in the office. Mornings can be hectic, and some people might find it easier to default to standard work attire rather than taking the time to put together an outfit that reflects their personal style. The pressure to adhere to a tight schedule can make it challenging to experiment with different looks.

The workplace culture and atmosphere can impact how individuals approach personal style. In environments where conformity is highly valued, employees might feel discouraged from standing out or being too adventurous with their fashion choices. This can lead to a reluctance to express one's true self through clothing.

Another factor is the constant evolution of fashion trends. Keeping up with the latest styles while maintaining a personal style that aligns with one's preferences can be demanding. It requires a certain level of effort and awareness to adapt one's style to the latest trends without losing a sense of identity.

Despite these challenges, finding ways to incorporate elements of personal style into work attire can be rewarding. Whether it's through accessories, subtle touches, or mixing classic pieces with trendy items, expressing individuality can enhance confidence and foster a sense of authenticity in a professional setting. Dressing for work while considering your personal style can be a delightful blend of professionalism and self-expression. It's like finding the perfect balance between being a boss and being yourself! Embrace your unique fashion choices, and remember, you're not just dressing for success.

Personal style plays a crucial role in building confidence and self-esteem. Wearing outfits that make us feel good about ourselves and align with our self-perception can boost our confidence levels at work. When we feel empowered and comfortable in our clothing, we are more likely to face challenges with a positive mindset and greater resilience.

Assess your workplace's dress code and guidelines. Whether it's business formal, business casual, or somewhere in between, there's always room to add your personal touch. Just like your outfit, it should be polished, well-organised, and leave a lasting impression! Choose looks that make you feel confident and comfortable. After all, your clothing should never make you feel like you're stuck in a never-ending spreadsheet! Just like a software update, refresh your work wardrobe from time to time to keep it exciting and up-to-date. Add a new blouse, a stylish blazer, or a pair of sleek shoes to your repertoire (of course in line with your personal style), and watch your confidence soar higher than your inbox on Monday mornings!

Activity 9

While the primary focus should be abiding by your work dress code, write down ways in which you can incorporate your personal style at work. Consider accessories, subtle touches, your bag, or your shoe choice to express individuality.

Dressing in your personal style for specific events can be challenging due to various factors that come into play during event dressing. Many events come with specific dress codes that participants are expected to follow. These dress codes might dictate formal attire, black tie, cocktail attire, or business casual, limiting your freedom to express your personal style fully. Adhering to the dress code can lead to a more standardised and uniform appearance, making it difficult to showcase your unique fashion preferences.

Depending on the event, there might be social expectations to dress a certain way to fit in or meet the perceived norms of the occasion. The fear of standing out or being judged can influence your clothing choices, potentially pushing you to conform rather than embrace your personal style.

Dressing for events can sometimes trigger feelings of insecurity or self-consciousness. You might question whether your personal style is appropriate for the occasion, or if it will be well-received by others. This can lead to second-guessing and opting for safer, more conventional clothing choices instead of staying true to your unique style.

In some cases, your existing wardrobe might not align perfectly with the event's theme or dress code. Finding suitable pieces that both resonate with your personal style and meet the event's requirements can be challenging, especially if time and budget constraints come into play.

Special events often come with the desire to make a lasting impression. This pressure to "dress to impress" can override your usual personal style choices, as you may feel compelled to opt for more eye-catching or attention-grabbing outfits that deviate from your everyday look. Dressing for certain events might be unfamiliar territory for some individuals. A lack of experience in event dressing can lead to uncertainty about what's appropriate or how to strike a balance between personal style and event requirements.

Dressing in your personal style for events can be challenging due to dress code restrictions, social expectations, insecurity, wardrobe limitations, pressure to impress, and unfamiliarity with event dressing. However, it's essential to strike a balance that allows you to incorporate elements of your personal style while also respecting the event's requirements. The key is to strike a balance between honouring the occasion's dress code and staying true to your unique fashion preferences.

Start by understanding the event's theme and dress code. Whether it's a formal gala, a casual gathering, or a themed party, knowing the expectations will help you navigate your outfit choices. But don't be afraid to add your personal twist to the ensemble. For example, if it's a black-tie event, you can opt for a classic gown or a tailored suit that reflects your style, accessorising with statement pieces that add a touch of flair.

Consider the colours and silhouettes that you feel most comfortable and confident in. If bright and bold hues make you feel alive, incorporate them into your outfit. If you prefer a more subdued palette, focus on elegant neutrals that still make a statement. The key is to feel like the best version of yourself while exuding charisma and charm.

Accessories play a crucial role in event dressing. They offer an excellent opportunity to add personal touches to your outfit. Whether it's a unique necklace, a vintage clutch, or eye-catching shoes, these accessories can reflect your interests and passions. Remember, fashion is an art form, and accessorising is like adding the finishing brushstrokes to a masterpiece.

As you curate your event outfit, consider the venue and the weather. Practicality doesn't mean compromising style. If the event is outdoors, opt for comfortable yet fashionable footwear and fabrics that suit the climate without sacrificing elegance.

Lastly, don't forget to embrace the joy of dressing up and have fun with it. Events are celebrations, and your outfit should reflect your excitement. Dressing for an event is an opportunity to express yourself, show off your creativity, and make a lasting impression, all while staying true to your personal style. So, go ahead and rock that event with your unique flair, leaving a lasting impression on everyone around you.

Activity 10

You probably have an event coming up in your diary. When you plan your outfit for your next event, ensure you have two key elements of personal style. This could be your shoes and bag. And most importantly, make sure that you feel comfortable!

8

Your Body Shape

If you often find yourself wondering, "What is my body type?" we have you covered. We understand the frustration of picking the perfect dress while shopping, only to be disappointed when it doesn't fit as expected in the trial room. Often, this disappointment stems from a lack of awareness about different body types. However, once you become familiar with your own body structure, showcasing your dream outfit becomes a reality. Therefore, it is essential to learn about the different body types and identify which one you belong to for a more enjoyable and successful shopping experience.

Understanding your body type is essential for dressing well because it helps you choose clothes that complement your figure and accentuate your best features. Each body type has distinct proportions and shapes, and certain clothing styles may flatter one body type more than another. When you know your body type, you can select clothes that enhance your natural curves and minimise any areas you might not feel as confident about.

For example, if you have an hourglass body shape characterised by a well-defined waist and balanced proportions between your bust and hips, you can opt for clothing that emphasises your waist, such as fitted dresses, belted tops, and high-waisted bottoms. On the other hand, if you have a pear-shaped

47

body with wider hips and a narrower waist and shoulders, you might want to draw attention to your upper body by wearing statement tops or jackets while choosing bottoms that create a balanced silhouette. We will cover all the body shapes later on!

Knowing your body type can also make shopping for clothes a more enjoyable and successful experience. By understanding the styles that suit your body shape, you can avoid trying on clothes that are unlikely to be flattering, saving time and frustration. You'll be able to focus on pieces that you know will make you look and feel great, making your wardrobe more cohesive and functional.

Furthermore, being aware of your body type promotes body confidence and self-acceptance. No body type is inherently superior to another; each has its own unique beauty. By understanding that different body shapes are natural variations, you can appreciate and embrace your body for what it is rather than striving for an unrealistic and idealised body standard.

Knowing your body type is crucial for dressing well because it enables you to make informed fashion choices that enhance your appearance and confidence. Embracing your body shape and wearing clothes that highlight your best features can empower you to feel more comfortable and content in your own skin. Dressing for your body type is not about conforming to societal standards but rather about celebrating your individuality and expressing your personal style with confidence.

Activity 11

Before delving into understanding your body type and dressing accordingly, it is essential to know your measurements accurately. Taking your measurements provides a solid foundation for finding clothes that fit you perfectly.

Using a cloth tape measure is preferable to a metal one, as it conforms better to your body's contours and ensures more accurate results.

When measuring, be sure not to make the tape too tight or too loose. It should be snug around the areas you are measuring, just enough that you think it might slip. Don't worry if it does slip a bit; simply hold onto it firmly to get the most precise measurement possible. Taking measurements in this manner will allow you to confidently select clothing sizes and styles that flatter your figure and make you feel comfortable and confident.

By combining an understanding of your body type with accurate measurements, you can approach shopping and dressing with greater confidence and ease. You'll be equipped with the knowledge to choose clothes that enhance your best features and fit like a dream, making your fashion choices truly tailored to your unique body shape and size.

Jot down your measurements for your shoulders, bust, waist, and hips in your note book.

Shoulder measurements: Obtaining accurate shoulder measurements can be a bit challenging, as it requires keeping the tape in place while measuring. If you find it tricky to manage on your own, consider enlisting the help of someone else, especially if there are people around who can assist you. To measure your shoulders, start at the tip of one shoulder, then bring the tape around to the other side until it meets the tip of the same shoulder again. Ensure that the tape is positioned very close to the shoulder for precise results. This method allows you to accurately determine the measurement of the widest point of your shoulders. With this crucial measurement, you'll have a better understanding of how clothing and accessories will fit across your shoulders, helping you make more informed fashion choices.

Bust measurements: Before taking the bust measurement, stand straight with good posture. Begin by locating the fullest part of your bust, and then position one end of the tape measure at this point. Gently wrap the tape around your body, starting from under your shoulders and bringing it back to where you started. Be careful not to compress your breasts with the tape; it should lie smoothly against your chest from end to end. This way, you can obtain an accurate measurement of your bust size, which will be invaluable when choosing tops, dresses, and bras that fit you perfectly and comfortably. If you are someone who likes to wear clothes below your belly button as part of their personal style, you might want to make a note of that number too.

Waist measurements: Maintain an upright posture without slouching or pulling in your stomach. Stand as straight as possible. To measure your waist accurately, identify the slimmest part of your midsection, located above your belly button and below the rib cage; this is your natural waistline.

Hip measurements: To measure your hips accurately, determine the circumference of the fullest part of your buttocks. Begin by placing the tape measure on one side of your hip and wrapping it around to the other hip, passing through the rear. Bring the tape back to the starting point to complete the measurement. It's advisable to perform this exercise in front of a mirror to ensure that the tape remains level and aligned throughout the process. By doing so, you'll obtain a precise hip measurement, which will aid you in selecting bottoms and dresses that fit comfortably and flatter your unique body shape.

By identifying your body type, you can map out the most flattering clothing choices and tailor them to suit your unique style. The goal is to select pieces that sit beautifully and proportionately on your body, creating a more balanced and appealing silhouette.

Contrary to popular belief, body types are not solely determined by height, weight, or specific measurements. Instead, they depend on the overall shape and distribution of body parts. Whether you're short, tall, slender, curvy, or somewhere in between, the focus is on the proportions and contours of your body.

Although each person's body shape is distinct, they typically fall into broader categories or body type "buckets." By understanding these general categories, you can delve deeper into identifying your specific body type and what works best for you. Embracing your body type and dressing according to its proportions will ensure that you look and feel your best in any outfit.

So let's break down the different body shapes and how to dress for each.

Apple body shape: The apple body shape, also known as the oval-shaped figure, is characterised by having a heavier upper body in comparison to the lower part. Individuals with this body type typically have broad shoulders, a larger bust line, and an appearance of weight gathering around the midriff.

Dressing for an apple body shape involves taking attention away from the midriff, which tends to appear heavier due to the concentration of weight above the hips and a less defined waistline. The key is to highlight your strengths and create the illusion of an elongated torso. To achieve this, consider flaunting your legs with skirts or dresses that hit above the knee. Additionally, opt for V or deep V necklines, which draw the eyes upward and elongate the upper body, diverting attention from the midsection. By strategically choosing these styles, you can enhance your overall appearance and feel more confident in your outfits.

Accentuating the face with accessories like necklaces and earrings can be a smart way to divert attention from the heavier midsection. Additionally, showcasing your legs through well-chosen skirts or dresses and stylish footwear can create a balanced and flattering look, shifting the focus away from the midriff and enhancing overall confidence in fashion choices.

A-line or empire cuts are ideal choices, providing a flattering silhouette.

Opt for printed dresses, patterned jackets, or flowy tops that add layers to the outfit. Monochrome looks and dark colours work well, as do full or 3/4-sleeve dresses. Flared bottoms and palazzo pants can create a balanced appearance. Given the broader shoulders and potentially larger bustline, it's crucial to wear the right bra for proper support and comfort (we will dive into all things underwear later on).

To flatter the apple body shape, steer clear of figure-hugging dresses or tops paired with skinny jeans, as they can emphasise the midsection. Instead, opt for looser-fitting clothing to create a more balanced look. Consider using an upper waist belt rather than a regular waist belt to maintain proportions. Waistband trousers and skirts with elastic bands are excellent choices for this body shape, providing both comfort and style.

Hourglass shape: The hourglass body shape is characterised by a well-defined waist where the bust and hips are approximately the same width, creating a balanced and curvaceous silhouette. Women with an hourglass figure typically have fuller busts, rounded hips, and a narrow waistline, giving the appearance of an hourglass-like outline. This body shape is often considered the most coveted and classic, as it naturally exhibits feminine curves. Dressing for the hourglass body shape involves highlighting the waist and choosing clothing that accentuates the curves while maintaining a balanced and proportionate appearance.

Dressing for an hourglass body shape involves celebrating your well-balanced figure by choosing clothing styles that complement and accentuate your curves. Embrace the natural beauty of your silhouette by opting for dresses that fit perfectly in the right places, following the outline of your curves. Take advantage of this coveted body shape and showcase your feminine proportions with pride. Emphasise your defined waist and select clothing that highlights your bust and hips, creating a harmonious and proportional look that accentuates your unique curves.

The best clothes for an hourglass body shape are dresses that cinch at the waist, as they highlight and enhance your well-defined waistline. V or plunge V necklines and sweetheart necklines are perfect for showcasing your upper body and accentuating your bust. To further flaunt your waistline, opt for a belt positioned at your natural waist or slightly below the belly button; either way, it looks fantastic. A-line dresses or similar cuts are excellent choices for the lower part of your body, as they create a balanced and flattering silhouette. Additionally, don't shy away from body-hugging dresses that accentuate your curves, as they are made for your figure and exude confidence and elegance. Embrace your hourglass shape and enjoy dressing in styles that celebrate your beautiful proportions.

While an hourglass body shape looks great in almost anything, it's essential to avoid pairing it with loose tops or bottoms, as they can potentially disrupt the balanced and flattering silhouette. Loose-fitting clothing may hide the natural curves and proportions that define the hourglass figure, which could detract from the natural curves of this figure. Instead, opt for styles that accentuate your waist, and these curves, as well-fitted clothing will highlight your best features and showcase your beautiful figure with confidence and grace. Embrace your shape and choose outfits that ensure that your hourglass body remains the centre of attention in any ensemble.

Pear shape: The pear body shape is characterised by having a narrower upper body and wider hips and thighs, resembling the shape of a pear. Women with a pear body shape typically have a smaller bust, a defined waist, and fullness in the hips, buttocks, and thighs. This body type tends to carry more weight in the lower half of the body, while the upper body remains relatively slender. Dressing for a pear body shape involves balancing the proportions by highlighting the upper body and waist while minimising emphasis on the hips and thighs. The goal is to create a more balanced silhouette and showcase the natural curves in a flattering manner.

Dressing for a pear body shape involves creating the illusion of an hourglass figure by balancing the proportions between the narrower upper body and wider hips. To achieve this, focus on enhancing the lower body or striking a balance between the upper and lower parts. Opt for clothing that draws attention upward, such as tops with interesting necklines, statement sleeves, or eye-catching patterns. This will highlight your shoulders and upper body. Additionally, choose bottoms that flatter your hips and thighs, like A-line skirts, bootcut or wide-leg pants, and dark-coloured bottoms. By emphasising your lower body or finding the right balance, you can showcase your beautiful curves and feel confident in your fashion choices.

Skinny jeans paired with loose tops can also help create an hourglass illusion by drawing attention upward. Additionally, consider wearing crop tops, sweetheart, V, or deep-V necklines, padded jackets, scoop, or boat necks to add volume and balance to the upper body, taking the focus away from the hips. Embrace these styles to enhance your pear-shaped figure and feel confident and stylish in your clothing choices.

When you have a pear-shaped body, it's best to avoid certain clothing styles that might not flatter your proportions. Steer clear of skin-fitting tops, as they can emphasise the contrast between your narrower upper body and wider hips, drawing too much attention to the lower half. Halter necklines may also accentuate the shoulders, further highlighting the difference between the upper and lower body. Moreover, loose bottoms can add bulk to the hip area, potentially making it appear larger. However, if you prefer these looks, don't hesitate to wear them. The key is to find a balance that complements your body shape and makes you feel confident and beautiful in your outfit choices.

Rectangle Shape: A rectangular body shape, also known as a straight body or banana body shape, is characterised by having relatively equal measurements in the bust, waist, and hips. This body shape typically lacks pronounced curves, creating a straight and elongated silhouette. The waist is not as defined as in other body types, and the overall appearance is more angular and athletic. With a rectangular body shape, the goal of dressing is often to create the illusion of curves and add more definition to the waistline.

When dressing for a rectangle body shape, focus on accentuating your assets, which are your arms and legs. While your body shape may resemble an hourglass figure without a defined waistline, the goal is to create the illusion of curves and add more definition to your silhouette. Opt for sleeveless tops, off-the-shoulder styles, or dresses with shorter hemlines to highlight your arms and legs. A-line skirts and dresses with belts or cinched waistbands can also help add shape to your figure. Layering with jackets or tops can add volume and create the appearance of curves. Embrace your unique body shape and experiment with different styles to find what makes you feel confident and stylish.

For a rectangle-shaped body, the best clothes are those that add curves and definition to your figure. Opt for A-line skirts and dresses that create the illusion of a more defined waistline. Ruffled and layered tops can add volume and shape to your upper body. Choose dresses with details or patterns that enhance your bottom and necklines like sleeveless, strapless, or sweetheart lines that add fullness to the upper body. Blazers, long jackets, and capes can add much-needed drama and structure to your silhouette.

It's best to avoid dresses that are overly voluminous or overarching, as they can overwhelm your figure and create a boxy appearance. Such dresses may look consuming and not flatter your body shape. Avoid shapeless or baggy clothing that hides your natural proportions, as they may not showcase your best features.

Inverted Triangle: An inverted triangle body shape is characterised by having broader shoulders and bust compared to the hips and waist, resembling an upside-down triangle. This body type typically features a wider upper body with well-defined shoulders, a full bust, and a narrower waist and hips. The hips and thighs are generally more slender in proportion to the shoulders and upper body.

Dressing for an inverted triangle body shape involves balancing the proportions by drawing attention away from the broad shoulders and enhancing the lower body to create a more balanced and flattering silhouette. A great way to do this is by adding definition to the hips. Opt for straight-cut jeans and dresses that naturally have an inverted V-look, as they can help create the illusion of wider hips and a more proportional figure. A-line skirts and dresses can also flatter your shape by balancing the broader upper body with the lower body. Choose tops with lower necklines, such as V-necks or scoop necks, to draw attention downward and away from the shoulders. Additionally, consider layering with jackets or cardigans that hit the hips to add volume to the lower body. Embrace these styles to enhance your inverted triangle body shape and feel confident and stylish in your clothing choices.

The best clothes are those that balance broader shoulders with narrower hips. Pencil-cut skirts and skinny jeans paired with any top will look great, as they emphasise the hips and create a more proportional silhouette. Avoid excessive layering or adding definition to the upper body, as it's already well-defined. Instead, opt for tops with lower necklines, such as V-necks or scoop necks, to draw attention downward and create a more balanced look. Embrace these styles to enhance your inverted triangle body shape and feel confident in your looks.

It's best to avoid wearing excessive patterns, ruffles, and layers on the upper body. Instead, let these elements be part of the bottom part of your body, such as A-line skirts or dresses with interesting details. Keep the upper body minimalistic and opt for simple and clean-cut tops to draw attention away from the broad shoulders and create a more balanced look. Embrace this approach, and you will not only look great but also enhance your shape.

Activity 12

Using your measurements, identify which body shape you are and create three outfits using pieces from your current wardrobe to complement your body shape. Take pictures of these looks to refer to in the future when you are in need of some outfit inspiration.

Gone are the days of feeling disappointed or insecure when wearing your dream outfit, only to find it doesn't look as great as you expected. Now that you understand the underlying reasons behind feeling uncomfortable in certain clothes that may look perfect on others, it's not about trying to emulate mannequins or influencers, but rather about dressing according to your unique body type and fashion sense. By doing so, you'll emphasise your best features. Dressing in a way that makes you feel confident and comfortable in your own skin is what truly matters.

Knowing your body shape is essential for perfecting your personal style, as it enables you to make informed and flattering fashion choices that enhance your natural features and highlight your best assets. Each body shape has its own unique proportions, and understanding yours allows you to select clothing that complements your silhouette, creating a harmonious and visually appealing look.

Identifying your body shape helps you find clothing that fits well. Ill-fitting garments can make you feel uncomfortable and self-conscious, whereas clothes that are tailored to your body shape will drape elegantly and enhance your overall appearance. By knowing your body shape, you can focus on styles, cuts, and fabrics that flatter your figure, resulting in a more polished and put-together ensemble.

Secondly, it saves you time and effort while shopping. With so many fashion choices available, it's easy to feel overwhelmed. Knowing your body shape narrows down the options, allowing you to concentrate on pieces that are likely to look great on you. This not only simplifies the shopping process but also reduces the likelihood of purchasing items that will end up sitting unused in your closet.

Understanding your body shape empowers you to embrace and celebrate your unique attributes. By recognising what makes your body distinctive, you can develop a positive body image and feel more confident in your appearance. Embracing body positivity means recognising that there is no single "ideal" body shape and that every shape is beautiful in its own way. Your personal style becomes a reflection of your individuality and self-acceptance.

Knowing your body shape is a fundamental aspect of perfecting your personal style. It not only ensures that your clothing fits well and saves you time while shopping, but it also fosters body positivity and empowers you to embrace your uniqueness. By dressing in a way that complements your figure, you can confidently showcase your personal style and radiate self-assurance in every outfit you wear. Remember, fashion is not about conforming but about celebrating your own beauty and authenticity.

9

Considering Sustainability

In today's world, it would be wrong to discuss fashion without mentioning some of the negative impacts of fast fashion and the importance of sustainability. The link between sustainability, personal style, and well-being is a powerful connection that highlights how our fashion choices can profoundly impact both ourselves and the environment. Embracing sustainable fashion practises goes beyond simply following trends; it involves making mindful decisions about the clothing we wear and the way we present ourselves to the world.

Being sustainable and fashionable can present challenges due to various factors that intersect within the fashion industry and consumer behaviour. There are many reasons why it might be difficult to balance sustainability and getting your fashion fix.

Firstly, fast fashion promotes the rapid production of trendy and inexpensive clothing, leading to overconsumption and a constant need for new styles. This culture encourages disposable fashion, making it challenging for sustainable brands to compete with the low prices and frequent releases of fast fashion retailers. Unless you have been living under a rock, I am sure you have watched a horrendous documentary about some of the quickly growing fast fashion brands. One of the popular fast fashion brands leaves about 6.3

million tonnes of carbon dioxide a year in its trail—a number that falls well below the 45% target to reduce global carbon emissions by 2030, which the U.N. has said is necessary for fashion companies to implement to help limit global warming. To make matters worse, the workers in most of these fast fashion factories were working up to 18-hour days and were given only one day off a month. In the factory of one of the most famous fast fashion brands, the outlet found women washing their hair during lunch breaks. In addition to this, these workers were then fined 2/3 of their daily pay if they made a mistake on a piece of clothing. No one should have to work in these conditions. The pressure to keep up with rapidly changing fashion trends can drive consumers towards fast fashion. The desire to fit in and look "on-trend" can sometimes override the consideration of sustainability. It is so important to think twice when purchasing fast fashion—is it really worth it?

Many consumers may not be aware of the environmental and social impacts of their clothing choices. Without sufficient knowledge about sustainable fashion options, individuals may default to conventional and less eco-friendly choices. In some regions, access to sustainable fashion brands and stores might be limited. Consumers may find it challenging to discover sustainable options, especially in areas dominated by fast-fashion retailers. Sustainable and ethically produced clothing often comes with a higher price tag due to the use of eco-friendly materials, ethical labour practises, and smaller production runs. This higher cost can deter some consumers from choosing sustainable options. Some brands engage in greenwashing, using deceptive marketing to present themselves as more sustainable than they actually are. This can confuse consumers and make it difficult to discern genuinely sustainable options. Sustainable brands may have a narrower range of sizes and style options compared to mainstream fashion retailers. This can be a barrier for individuals with diverse fashion preferences and body types. Shifting consumer attitudes and habits towards sustainability can be challenging. Breaking away from the "more is better" mentality and embracing a slower, more conscious approach to fashion requires a change in mindset.

Despite these challenges, there is a growing movement towards sustainable fashion as consumers and brands increasingly recognise the importance of ethical and environmentally responsible choices. As sustainable practises become more mainstream, the fashion industry is gradually evolving to cater to the demands of conscious consumers. By raising awareness, making informed choices, and supporting sustainable brands, individuals can play a crucial role in pushing the fashion industry towards a more sustainable and fashion-forward future. By choosing sustainable clothing options, we contribute to reducing the environmental footprint of the fashion industry, which is notorious for its significant impact on natural resources and the climate. This alignment with sustainability in our personal style allows us to feel a deeper sense of purpose, knowing that our fashion choices are in harmony with our values of protecting the planet for future generations.

When we align our personal style with sustainability, we are also more likely to opt for quality over quantity. Sustainable fashion often emphasises timeless and durable pieces that are designed to last, reducing the need for constant replacements and curbing excessive consumerism. As a result, we can experience a greater sense of satisfaction and contentment with a smaller, curated wardrobe that reflects our true style identity.

Embracing sustainable fashion can lead to increased creativity and self-expression. Sustainable options often encourage repurposing and upcycling clothing items, allowing us to experiment with unique looks and styles. This creative freedom fosters a more authentic representation of our individuality, boosting our confidence and self-esteem.

In addition to its positive impact on the environment and personal style, sustainable fashion can enhance our overall well-being. By consciously choosing clothing that aligns with our values and beliefs, we establish a deeper connection between our inner selves and our outward appearance. This sense of coherence can promote a stronger sense of self-awareness and a more positive body image. Furthermore, supporting ethical and sustainable fashion brands can create a sense of community and connection with like-minded individuals. Engaging with sustainable fashion communities fosters a sense of belonging and shared purpose, which can contribute to overall happiness and mental well-being.

Embracing sustainable fashion practises empowers us to make mindful decisions about our clothing choices, reduce our environmental impact, and express our individuality in a more authentic way. By aligning our personal style with sustainability, we not only contribute to a healthier planet but also enhance our overall well-being by fostering a deeper sense of purpose, self-expression, and connection to like-minded communities.

Activity 13

There are many ways in which you can live a sustainable and fashionable lifestyle. Choose three of the following to incorporate into your life going forward in order to have a positive and sustainable impact:

Choose Quality Over Quantity: Invest in high-quality clothing and accessories that are designed to last. Opt for durable materials and timeless designs that won't go out of style quickly, reducing the need for frequent replacements.

Embrace Secondhand Shopping: Explore thrift stores, consignment shops, and online platforms for pre-loved clothing. Secondhand shopping allows you to find unique pieces and give existing clothing a new life, reducing the demand for fast fashion.

Support Sustainable Brands: Look for fashion brands that prioritise sustainability in their production processes, use eco-friendly materials, and have transparent ethical practises. Supporting such brands encourages the growth of sustainable fashion and sends a message to the industry.

Go for Versatility: Choose clothing that can be mixed and matched to create multiple outfits. Versatile pieces allow you to maximise your wardrobe without needing an excessive number of items.

Timeless Classics: Incorporating classic and timeless pieces into your wardrobe that won't be affected by short-lived trends, will then remain relevant year after year, so you don't have to buy as often.

Eco-Friendly Materials: Seek out clothing made from sustainable materials, such as organic cotton, Tencel, hemp, bamboo, and recycled fabrics. These materials have a lower environmental impact than conventional ones.

Practise Mindful Consumption: Before making a purchase, ask yourself if you truly need the item and how often you will wear it. Avoid impulse buys and focus on acquiring pieces that align with your personal style and values.

Explore DIY and Upcycling: Get creative and consider DIY projects or upcycling old clothing to give it a fresh look or repurpose it into new items.

Care for Your Clothing: Extend the lifespan of your garments by following proper care instructions, such as washing them in cold water and air-drying when possible. Proper care helps reduce wear and tear and minimises the need for replacements.

Borrow or Swap: Consider borrowing or swapping clothing with friends or participating in clothing swap events. This allows you to enjoy new looks without buying new items.

Avoid Single-Use Fashion: Refrain from purchasing clothing for a specific occasion only. Instead, aim for pieces that can be worn in different settings and events.

Be Mindful of Accessories: Choose sustainable and ethically made accessories, such as bags, shoes, and jewellery, to complement your outfits.

By integrating these sustainable practises into your fashion choices, you can cultivate a stylish and environmentally conscious wardrobe that reflects your personal style while making a positive impact on the planet. Remember, small individual actions collectively contribute to significant positive change in the fashion industry and beyond.

10

The Power of Perfect Underwear

The foundation of a good outfit extends beyond the clothes themselves. While clothing may be the centrepiece of our attire, what lies beneath plays a crucial role in determining how the entire ensemble looks and feels on our body. Underestimated but essential, underwear acts as the backbone that creates the desired silhouette, providing support and structure to our outfits. When the undergarments are chosen wisely and fit perfectly, the rest of the outfit follows suit, enhancing its overall appearance.

Underwear drawers are often overlooked and neglected in comparison to our wardrobes. While it's true that clothes are more visible to others than what's underneath, the importance of underwear should not be underestimated. There is a reason why we wear them in addition to our clothes, and it's time to shed light on the significance of lingerie and make them a priority in our wardrobe choices.

To truly appreciate the value of underwear, we must first understand its historical significance and the reasons it became an integral part of our everyday attire. Beyond its aesthetic appeal, one of the primary reasons we wear underwear is for hygiene purposes. Acting as a barrier between our skin and outer clothing, underwear helps maintain cleanliness and reduces the risk of direct contact between our bodies and potentially abrasive fabrics.

Understanding the importance of the right underwear is key to dressing well. Each outfit may demand specific types of underclothes to achieve the desired look and feel. By being mindful of which outfits require different types of underwear, we can ensure that our wardrobe choices complement and accentuate our overall style. Whether it's seamless underwear to maintain comfort and eliminate visible lines or shaping undergarments to enhance certain areas, making informed decisions about our lingerie empowers us to wear clothes with confidence and ease.

Underwear has also played a pivotal role in shaping the way women's bodies are perceived and presented throughout history. From corsets that created coveted hourglass figures to modern-day push-up bras and shaping garments like Spanx, underwear has been instrumental in achieving the desired silhouette for different fashion eras. These foundational garments are responsible for shaping and enhancing our body contours, which, in turn, affect how our outer clothing fits and appears on the surface.

The significance of investing in quality and well-fitting underwear is so underrated. Wearing ill-fitting or worn-out undergarments can lead to discomfort, chafing, and even health issues. In addition, seeing your bra strap in an otherwise perfectly curated outfit can absolutely ruin the look. Choosing the right lingerie that complements your body shape can boost confidence and self-assurance. Underclothes that don't fit properly can lead to discomfort, bunching, or riding up, which may distract from the outfit's overall impact. Conversely, wearing underwear that suits our body shape and complements the outfit ensures a seamless and polished appearance, elevating the entire look.

Of course, sexy lingerie is not just for outward display or the pleasure of others; it can be a powerful tool for self-expression and empowerment. Embracing sensuous underwear that makes you feel beautiful and confident can positively impact your self-image. Celebrating your body and appreciating it for all its uniqueness can lead to a greater sense of self-love and acceptance, which will radiate outward in your interactions and relationships.

The choices we make in our underwear drawer are also an intimate reflection of our personal style and preferences. Just like outerwear, undergarments come in a plethora of designs, fabrics, and colours to suit individual tastes. Selecting lingerie that resonates with your personality allows you to infuse a touch of individuality and flair into your daily routine, reminding you that even the most private aspects of your life deserve attention and care. As we curate our wardrobes, it's crucial to pay equal attention to the selection of underwear. Just like we carefully choose our outer garments based on occasions and moods, considering the right lingerie for each outfit enhances the overall fashion experience. Whether it's a strapless bra for a formal gown or seamless pants for figure-hugging attire, these seemingly minor details can make a significant difference in how we feel and present ourselves.

Embracing the importance of underwear as an essential part of our wardrobe can lead to a shift in mindset regarding self-care and self-worth. The foundation of a good outfit lies not only in the clothes we wear but also in the right selection of underwear that supports and shapes our silhouette. Undergarments play a crucial role in enhancing the overall appearance, comfort, and confidence of our outfits. By understanding which types of underwear complement different ensembles and prioritising well-fitted, attractive lingerie, we can elevate our fashion choices and embrace a more holistic approach to dressing.

So, let's break down some underwear options:

Seamless boyshorts: This is an ideal choice for wearing under bodycon dresses, as they effectively eliminate the awkward panty lines that can ruin a sleek look. Moreover, the high-waisted design of this style of underwear not only ensures a smooth silhouette but also imparts a slimming effect when paired with tight dresses. For light-coloured dresses with sheer material, opting for a nude or white-coloured pair ensures discreet coverage and maintains the outfit's elegance and confidence.

Bikini briefs: These are the perfect choice to wear under skinny jeans, offering both comfort and practicality. Their design allows for easy stretching and movement when paired with tight-fitting jeans, and the absence of seams ensures a smooth appearance, preventing visible panty lines that could mar the overall look. Opting for bikini briefs made of thin cotton material adds to the comfort level, promotes better ventilation, and ensures a relaxed and pleasant experience throughout the day.

Thongs: These are the perfect choice for wearing under tight-fitting shorts or skirts due to their design and practicality. The higher cut of thongs ensures there are no visible panty lines, eliminating any concerns about underwear being longer than the clothes, which could be a distraction. In addition, when dealing with shorts that tend to ride up, the higher cut of thongs comes to the rescue, effectively concealing them and keeping your underwear hidden from view, allowing you to move with confidence and comfort throughout the day.

G-string: This is a must-have for any lady when it comes to wearing fitted garments that hug the body closely. When boyshorts and seamless underwear fall short of providing a smooth look, a G-string comes to the rescue. It's an essential addition to every woman's lingerie collection, ensuring that there are no unsightly panty lines beneath skin-tight clothing. G-strings offer just the right coverage while maintaining a discreet profile, making them the perfect choice to achieve a flawless appearance and feel confident in any outfit.

Cotton hipsters: This underwear choice makes an excellent everyday choice for several reasons. Their breathable nature allows air circulation, which effectively reduces the risk of odours and bacterial buildup, thereby preventing discomfort and infections. With their comfort, hygiene, and practicality, cotton hipster pants offer a reliable and convenient option for you to feel at ease and confident throughout your daily activities.

Underwear comes in various styles to suit various occasions and outfits. When shopping for new underwear, it's crucial to take accurate measurements to ensure optimal comfort. Knowing the right size and understanding your body's hip and waist measurements will help you choose the appropriate underwear size, guaranteeing a perfect fit and preventing any discomfort. Whether it's seamless boyshorts for bodycon dresses, bikini briefs for skinny jeans, or thongs for skin-tight attire, having the right measurements will empower you to make confident and informed choices, enhancing your overall comfort and confidence every day.

Activity 14

You have cleared out your wardrobe, but many of you would have looked over the underwear drawer. However, it is now time to see to the dreaded underwear drawer. Throw away any pieces that don't fit, are worn out, or are just simply uncomfortable. Once this is done, it is time to take yourself shopping (in person, NOT online) to an underwear store, book yourself in for a bra fitting to know your true size, and purchase any underwear garments you may need. Think both sexy and practical!

11

The Same Size But Fits Differently

If our shoes sizes don't change from shop to shop, why do our clothes? The frustration of inconsistent clothing sizes from one shop to another is a common experience for many. However, understanding the reasons behind these variations can shed light on why sizes differ and how brands approach their sizing decisions.

Our bodies are unique, and even if two individuals wear the same size, they can have different proportions and body shapes. This diversity makes it challenging for brands to establish a one-size-fits-all approach to clothing sizing. Brands typically have an ideal customer in mind, and their fit models represent the body type they are targeting. The measurements of these fit models serve as the basis for creating size charts and blocks to guide the production of various sizes.

As a result, different brands cater to different target customers, leading to variations in sizing between stores. For example, a size 10 in one store may fit differently from a size 10 in another store due to the distinct preferences and body shapes of their target customers.

Even within the same brand, size discrepancies can occur, especially in fast fashion companies, where the focus might be on releasing new styles quickly rather than perfecting the fit. In such cases, inconsistent sizing may arise, causing further frustration for us consumers.

The inconsistency in clothing sizes among different brands can have a negative impact on consumers for several reasons. First, it can lead to frustration and confusion. When shoppers encounter varying sizes in different stores, it becomes challenging to know which size to pick without trying on multiple options. This process can be time-consuming and disheartening, as it creates uncertainty about which size will fit best. As a result, the shopping experience becomes less enjoyable, and customers may become discouraged from making purchases.

Secondly, inconsistent sizing can trigger body image concerns. When individuals find that they need to go up a size in a particular brand compared to others, it may lead to feelings of inadequacy or self-consciousness. The focus on numerical sizing can cause individuals to fixate on their bodies' perceived flaws rather than appreciating their unique shapes and sizes. This negative self-perception can impact self-esteem, leading to a diminished sense of body confidence. When different brands follow different fit models and size charts, it perpetuates the notion that there is an "ideal" body shape or size. This can create pressure for individuals to conform to these standards, even if it means striving for a specific clothing size that may not align with their natural proportions.

The negative impact of inconsistent sizing extends to the environmental and economic aspects of the fashion industry. When consumers purchase multiple sizes to find the right fit, it can lead to a higher rate of returns, resulting in increased waste and environmental impact. Additionally, the need to try different sizes may lead to excessive consumption, as customers may buy more items than necessary to ensure they find the right fit, contributing to overconsumption and potential financial strain.

Overall, the inconsistency in clothing sizes can have a host of negative consequences for consumers. It can result in frustration, body image concerns, unrealistic beauty standards, and environmental and economic issues. As a solution, brands can strive for more standardised sizing practises or provide better sizing information and fit guidance to assist customers in finding the right fit. Some brands are now adopting innovative solutions to assist customers in finding their best fit. Online retailers like ASOS are using customer data and preferences to suggest suitable sizes based on previous purchases. While this approach is not foolproof, it offers a more tailored sizing experience and can be helpful for consumers seeking the right fit.

Ultimately, the key to a satisfying wardrobe lies in feeling confident and comfortable in the clothes we wear. Embracing the fact that our bodies are unique and may require different sizes from various brands can help us focus on finding clothes that make us feel good rather than being fixated on the number on the tag.

While finding a perfect solution to standardise clothing sizes across all brands may be challenging, acknowledging and appreciating our individuality can empower us to build a wardrobe that truly reflects our personal style and fits our bodies comfortably. As long as we feel confident and at ease in our clothing choices, the quest for the perfect size becomes less critical, and we can embrace the joy of fashion without the constraints of arbitrary numbers.

Activity 15

Going forward, add a notes page to your phone where you can jot down the size you are in different brands. Of course, consider different types of garments like tops and trousers, as these will most likely be different sizes too. You can then refer to this in the future when you are shopping online or when you simply cannot be bothered to try on lines in the changing room. However, keep in mind that sizes may change from piece to piece within one retailer, so this hack may not always work.

12

Final Thoughts

Style can be a curious aspect of our lives. For years, we might feel completely content and confident in the outfits we put together without a second thought. But suddenly, there comes a day when we wake up and discover that our confidence has vanished, and we can't seem to find that same sense of self we once had. While clothing has the remarkable ability to instantly transform us, empower us, and create connections, it can also lead to confusion. Figuring out what message we want to convey with our clothes, how we desire to feel when we wear them, and who we aspire to be becomes a daunting task. The fashion industry, a vast multi-billion-dollar global business, offers countless job opportunities and livelihoods, ranging from technology and garment production to designers, models, and content creators. However, despite its significance, fashion is sometimes dismissed as a superficial, unintellectual realm not worthy of serious discussion. Yet, the impact our wardrobe can have on our emotions and self-perception is substantial, influencing the difference between feeling dreary or happy. Fashion can be a therapeutic journey of self-discovery, where experimentation and embracing what doesn't work are essential steps towards understanding what truly resonates with us.

True happiness does not hinge on whether you are highly Instagrammed or if you can afford to indulge in designer bags every season. It runs much deeper than material possessions. Imposter syndrome is a genuine struggle when it comes to dressing, and merely wearing an outfit without feeling its impact means the clothes are wearing you rather than the other way around. Discovering your true self can be challenging; many seek security in emulating others or adopting trendy looks deemed 'in'. However, genuine comfort in your identity is reflected in the clothes that you wear, and true happiness lies in embracing an authentic and self-assured style.

As humans, we often seek guidelines to aid in decision-making, enabling us to narrow down our choices and avoid the overwhelming paradox of too many options (of which there are many within the fashion world). Otherwise, we might end up feeling unsatisfied and lost. The activities within this book are designed to assist you in refining your personal style by providing the means to explore and discover your true preferences and create a sense of fulfilment in yourself throughout your fashion journey.

By working through each activity, you should have learned a lot about yourself and your personal style, as well as transformed your wardrobe for the better. But it doesn't stop here; continue exploring your own personal style by experimenting with different clothing choices. Don't be afraid to pick up this book in the future and take yourself through each activity again. This process of self-discovery will contribute to more authentic self-expression through fashion.

Discuss what you have learned with your friends and create conversations around personal style. This will create a supportive and inspiring environment where everyone can learn, grow, and celebrate their unique fashion journeys together. By engaging in these conversations, you can help boost each other's confidence and reinforce the belief that fashion is not just about appearance but a powerful means of self-expression.

Fashion can be surprisingly therapeutic, providing a delightful and fun way to lift our spirits. Don't underestimate its power! Putting together a fabulous outfit can be a great way to lift your mood. When we're feeling down, retail therapy can be the perfect antidote (within our means, of course). There's something magically uplifting about finding that perfect dress or pair of shoes that just speaks to us. Even if it's just for a moment, slipping into a new outfit can transport us to a world of confidence, which can be such a powerful tool to be aware of.

Remember, fashion is meant to be exciting and reflective of who you are. By embracing playfulness, creativity, and a positive attitude towards your wardrobe, you continue to evolve your style in exciting ways, which can help you feel like the best version of yourself.

13

Extras

Dear Reader,

I hope you've enjoyed getting to know your personal style. The stunning looks are just starting, and I can't wait for your style to evolve. I hope you enjoyed the book and drop a quick review where ever you made your purchase. Thank you and happy reading!

In addition to this, I have managed to get access for you to sign up for a fashion newsletter where you can get the latest trends straight into your inbox. Simply scan the QR code.

Also, keep your eyes out for my men's styling book which may be a great gift for the guys in your life that may need a hand with their wardrobe & how to dress.

Tara x